YOGA FOR BEGINNERS

Your Personal Journey to Health and Happiness

Disclaimer and Terms of Use:

Effort has been made to ensure that the information in this book is accurate and complete, however, the author and the publisher do not warrant the accuracy of the information, text and graphics contained within the book due to the rapidly changing nature of science, research, known and unknown facts and internet. The Author and the publisher do not hold any responsibility for errors, omissions or contrary interpretation of the subject matter herein. This book is presented solely for motivational and informational purposes only.

Table of Contents

Introduction

Yoga is a wonderful way to transform your life. There is no need to wait to start practicing yoga. You can begin your own practice today. This book's intention is to enlighten the reader on how to begin their very own yoga practice through information about the history, philosophy, physical practice, and meditation aspects of yoga.

You may assume that yoga is only for a certain kind of people, but the truth is that yoga is for everyone. Sure, there are many photos out there of people doing incredibly complex postures standing on their heads or putting a leg behind their head, but these are not necessary to truly do yoga. You have to remember that everyone is a beginner once. Yoga is meant to be a method of personal self-exploration for you, physically, mentally, and spiritually. The first thing is to realize that yoga can be practiced by anyone, anywhere, and at any time. Yoga is the perfect complement to any lifestyle.

If you feel intimidated by attending a yoga class in a group setting, it can be helpful to prepare yourself in advance. This manual will provide the knowledge and tools you need to start your own practice and step into a beginner's yoga class with ease whenever you are ready.

First, we will review what yoga is. We will outline the history of yoga and discuss the many different branches. Then, we will focus on the basics of the yoga poses essential for beginners to know. These poses will then be linked together into a simple sequence that you can practice on your own. Finally, we will discuss proper breathing and meditation techniques, as well as tips and advice on practicing yoga, advancing your practice, and finding the right class for you.

Why Do Yoga?

There are many reasons that people come to yoga or find the practice of yoga in their lives. You may seek peace of mind, ways to cope with your stress, or a method to lengthen and strengthen your body's muscles in a new way outside the old standard of weight lifting. Yoga has also been proven to benefit heart health, decrease insomnia, depression, anxiety, pain, and fatigue. It is also a positive way to increase the quality of life for cancer patients, and those living with asthma, high blood pressure, arthritis, and more.

If you are interested in learning yoga but do not feel ready to attend a public class yet, it is perfectly acceptable to begin practicing on your own. There are many valuable skills you can learn by teaching yourself something new. Often when you practice by yourself, there may also be fewer distractions. However, it is important to ensure that you understand what it is you are doing. If you have any injuries or health conditions, make note of these and speak with your doctor before starting a new regimen that could impact your physical well-being. Taking the time to learn on your own will also prepare you for the time you are ready to take a public yoga class.

Yoga in the western world is most often associated with stretching and flexibility. You do not need to be extremely flexible in order to do yoga. However, yoga is more than just merely stretching. Yoga incorporates deep breathing during the stretching postures and movements that bring fresh oxygen literally into your muscles and tissues. It is a mind-body practice that utilizes control of the breath as one of its most important principles.

Learning to utilize the mind body connection is essential to eliciting a relaxation response in the body. In today's world, we are overworked and likely suffering from not enough sleep, or perhaps we are eating the wrong things. When we learn to connect our mind to our body through yoga, meditation, and breathing techniques, we cannot only alleviate stress, but we can deal with challenging situations more efficiently. We can also help correct our attitudes, sleep patterns, and food habits to ones that are positive and healthy. Ultimately we all deserve a happy and nourished life. Yoga can help you accomplish that.

What is Yoga?

"Yoga is the joining or uniting of the mind, body and spirit to enrich the quality of one's life, and to enhance one's health."

Andrew Weil, M.D.

Yoga is an ancient science of physical, mental, and spiritual discipline that originated in India. It has its roots in Hindu philosophy as a means to achieve spiritual wisdom and peace through meditative practices. Many of its philosophical components are based on the Yoga Sutras of Patanjali.

Yoga is a Sanskrit word that means "to join". Essentially this means that yoga is a science of using the mind and body together to achieve a sense of unity.

Yoga philosophy and practice began to gain popularity in the western world in the 19th century with the first world tour of Swami Vivekananda. The 1960's are also widely regarded as a time when yoga became increasingly popular due to more interest in Eastern philosophy and the explosion of the pop band, The Beatles, and their study with gurus in India.

Many of today's most popular styles of yoga also originate from the work of Krishnamacharya, a prominent and influential yogi in the early 1900's. His students included B.K.S. Iyengar, Sri K. Pattahbi Jois, and TKV Desikachar, whom have each created their own unique style of yoga practice. Today the word "yoga" often refers to *hatha* yoga in the Western cultural setting, which is the practice of *asanas*, or postures. Yoga has proven to have a variety of positive connections to health in recent years, which has legitimized yoga as a form of purely physical exercise. This means that yoga is much more accessible than ever before.

The sage Patanjali is often referred to as the yogi who assembled yoga philosophy studied until now. Patanjali defines the word "yoga" in his second sutra, which is the definitional sutra for his entire work: "Yogash Chitta Vritti Nirodhah". It translates to "Yoga is restraining the mind-stuff (Chitta) from taking various forms (Vritti)".

Have you ever felt like you have too many thoughts going on inside your mind? It just so happens that this is a problem that not only many other people have, but that has been going on since the dawn of humankind. Yoga serves to quiet our minds through regular practice.

What are the Different Types of Yoga?

1. **Hatha Yoga**

   Hatha yoga is the most practiced type of yoga today. The Sanskrit roots of the word literally mean "sun" and "moon". This references the ability of the practice to bring together the energy of the sun and the moon in the body in working towards a balanced state. Hatha yoga is the physical side of yoga that utilizes postures with specific breathing techniques to cleanse and heal the body.

2. **Raja Yoga**

   This type of yoga is used for meditation purposes. Raja translates to "king" in Sanskrit; therefore, raja yoga is often referred to as "royal" yoga. Sages traditionally practice raja yoga.

3. **Jnana Yoga**

   This method of yoga focuses on learning and studying the ancient texts related to the practice. These texts include *The Bhagavad Gita*, *The Upanishads*, and *The Vedas.* Jnana translates to "wisdom" in Sanskrit. Its purpose is to develop the intellectual capacity of the practitioner.

4. **Karma Yoga**

   Karma yoga is the practice of selfless service. It is an act of altruism. Karma refers to how a person's decisions and actions will impact their future. For example, if you have a good attitude about life, you will have good karma. The opposite will be true if you have a bad attitude. It is the idea of practicing "you reap what you sow" in how you live your life. It is often displayed by helping others in need without being attached to the end results. In Sanskrit, the word karma comes from the prefix *kri*, which means "to do". Therefore, karma yoga is the practice of union through action.

5. Bhakti Yoga

Bhakti yoga is the yoga of devotion to a higher source of power, and is often practiced through kirtan. A kirtan is an energetic, call and response celebratory practice done in groups that sing mantras or devotional phrases and play instruments together. The practice of bhakti yoga is about channeling love of the divine as an active form of meditation. The word bhakti is derived from the Sanskrit root *bhaj*, which means "to worship".

What is a mantra?

A mantra is a transformative tool using words, sounds, or phrases. The most commonly used mantra in yoga is the sound of "OM". This sound is said to be the first vibration of the universe during its creation. It is often used at the beginning and/or end of a yoga class or session to reflect our existence in the universe.

Other Popular Mantras

There are many other mantras used in yoga practice as well. Another commonly used term is the word "Namaste". The teacher commonly uses this mantra at the end of a yoga class. It is an expression that means "I honor the light within you that is also within me." The Sanskrit interpretation of "Namaste" means "I bow to you". The mantra is used as a gesture of gratitude and respect between a teacher and their students by bringing the hands together in a prayer position at the heart, closing the eyes, saying the word, and bowing the head.

Another popular mantra is the phrase "lokah samastah sukhino bhavantu". Its interpretation is "may all beings be happy and free". It is commonly used in kirtan settings, or chanted by a teacher at the end of a session.

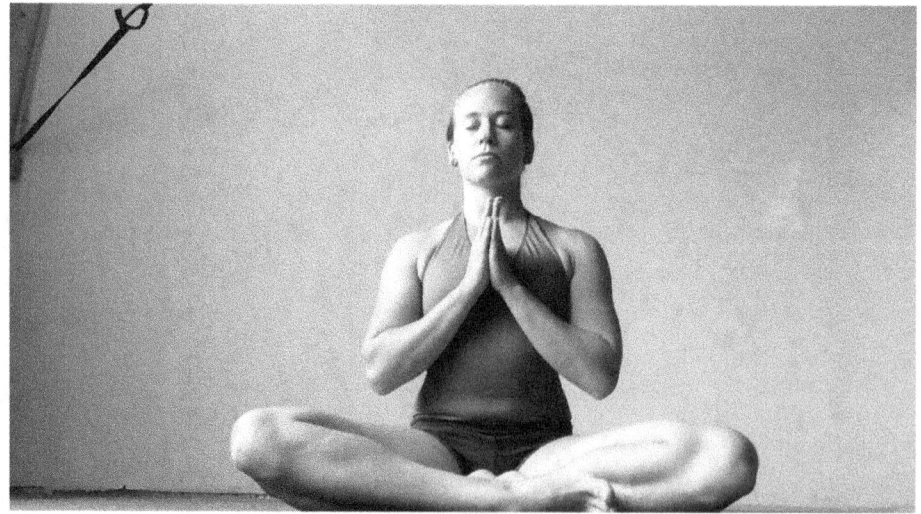

The Eight-Limbed Path of Yoga

Patanjali's writing also became the basis for a system referred to as Ashtanga Yoga, or Eight-Limbed Yoga. In brief the eight limbs, or steps to yoga, are as follows:

1. *Yama:* Universal morality
2. *Niyama:* Personal observances
3. *Asana:* Body postures (what most people practice in Western culture)
4. *Pranayama:* Breathing exercises, or control of prana (life force energy)
5. *Pratyahara:* Control of the senses
6. *Dharana:* Concentration and inner awareness
7. *Dhyana:* Devotion
8. *Samadhi:* Union

The first two limbs, *yamas* and *niyamas*, provide an ethical framework from which to live our lives. They help us to create personal morals and feelings that are inherently good, benefitting not only ourselves, but also all of life on our planet. They are suggestions on our attitudes and actions toward others and ourselves.

The *yamas* are divided into five characteristics. They outline our nature as caring, charitable, truthful, and peaceful. The *yamas* include:

1. *Ahimsa:* nonviolence
2. *Satya:* truthfulness
3. *Asteya:* nonstealing
4. *Brahmacharya:* abstinence or moderation
5. *Aparigraha:* noncovetousness

When following these guidelines, it becomes possible to integrate these principles as true life virtues. They help to purify our mental abilities and contribute to the goodness of society as a whole.

These universal morals are a guideline on how to live and interact with the world. The moment that we step onto our mats to practice, we enter into a state of truth- a place to be honest and sincere to our bodies and minds. We can use the physical postures of a yoga practice to be kind to ourselves, to explore new things, and to find our edges mentally and physically in a compassionate manner. We must practice *ahimsa* whenever we step onto our mats and be mindful of practicing something that may be physically dangerous and cause potential injury. Practicing moderation and being in the moment- and merely just wanting that. Not desiring what anyone else is doing, or even what the teacher is doing. We must embody our practice as ours alone, and love it for that.

The *niyamas* are personal observances that we as humans can make to become better people (at the very least). Ultimately following the *niyamas* will enhance our spiritual understanding and bring us closer to the Divine. The following are the *niyamas*:

1. **Saucha-** cleanliness
2. **Santosha-** contentment
3. **Tapas-** discipline
4. **Svadhyaya-** study of sacred scripture and of one's self
5. **Isvara pranidhana-** surrender to God

It is recommended to practice asana when one's body is in its most clean state. Physical yoga is essentially a detoxification process, so when we arrive to our mats physically clean, our practice will feel less toxic. Cultivating contentment during intense or seemingly slow moments of a practice is also an important facet to be aware of. It is not necessary to focus on all of these qualities at once or expect them to all happen at the same time. Often, you may find yourself dealing with individual *yamas* or *niyamas* head-on at different points in your practice. *Tapas* is the discipline of coming to the mat daily, to believing in yourself, and to doing that one last backbend even if you do not really feel like it. It keeps our inner fires burning just as much as each deep breath.

Svadhyaya and *isvara pranadhana* are much more internalized states of being. Eventually after much practice, we can use the tools of our bodies and minds for deep self-inquiry as we breathe, move, and hold postures on the mat. Ultimately, our intentions are to make each breath, movement, posture, and practice an offering or gift to God or a greater good so that we may experience more of the Divine in our daily lives. Though this spiritually charged movement practice may only occur for a certain amount of time each day, it has a magical way of seeping into every aspect of our lives so that we can live whole, connected, and joyful in every moment.

The practice of *asana* is the most familiar limb of yoga to most people. Asana involves the physical aspect of yoga. Asana can be translated to mean "staying still" or "comfortable seat". Traditionally, the practice of yoga postures is to prepare the body for meditation in a comfortable seated position. However, as the practice has progressed to include more advanced stretches and complicated poses, the philosophy of asana can be used as a tool to still the mind and find comfort in something that may be uncomfortable (but not painful). It can be used to open an inner awareness of the landscape of your body as well as a method to learn how to control your emotions and intentions to create a sense of unity between your body and mind. There are also many health benefits to practicing the physical side of yoga, which included increased flexibility, decreased pain, improved balance, coordination, strength, and overall wellness.

Pranayama is the practice of controlling your breath. Prana is translated as "life force energy". Our breath is the easiest method of connecting to this source of energy because it literally connects our internal and external worlds through respiration. Controlling prana through yoga is a way to promote and balance our physical and mental health and well-being.

Pranayama is often practiced after asana. The reason for this is because the asana has prepared the body to sit in a more balanced, comfortable, and controlled state. There are a few basic techniques that you can incorporate into your practice, although it is recommended to learn pranayama under an experienced teacher.

Ujjayi Breathing

Ujjayi breath is a breathing technique that you can actually use during asana. However, it helps to learn it by itself first. Ujjayi breath translates to "victorious" breath. This breathing technique creates a sense of power in the body and helps us to stay aligned with the breath when practicing.

Constricting the air in the back of the throat as you inhale and exhale, creating a slightly audible sound, activates this breathing technique. This sound will be reminiscent of a gentle ocean wave. Keeping your mouth closed, imagine that you can hum while inhaling and exhaling. By creating this audible sound, it also helps to encourage our awareness of the lengths of our breath, promoting balance from the very core of ourselves.

Alternate Nostril Breathing (Nadi Shodhana)

Alternate Nostril Breathing is another great technique that promotes balance in our body through controlling the breath. To perform this pranayama, follow these guidelines:

1. Sit comfortably and close your eyes
2. Place your left hand on your knee with the palm face up
3. Take your right hand and close your right nostril with the thumb
4. Inhale through the left side of your nose and then close the left side with your third and fourth fingers
5. Open the right nostril and exhale through that side.
6. Inhale through the right side and close with the thumb again.
7. Open the left nostril and exhale through the side.
8. Repeat each step.
9. Take at least 10 rounds, with each side equaling one set.

This technique allows you to take notice of any imbalances between the right and left sides of your body. It will also promote the balance of oxygen levels within the brain and help to clear the sinuses. It creates a calm response on the nervous system, alleviating any stress or concerns you may have.

The remaining four limbs of yoga are all concerned with the perception and control of the mind diving deeper into higher realms of consciousness. *Pratyahara* refers to the mind's ability to withdraw its senses from the external world to focus on the internal landscape. *Dharana* describes the pure mind control necessary for performing meditation and other activities. It is often referenced as finding *ekagrata*, or a single pointed focus. When *Dhyana* is fully experienced as an act or feeling of love, the person experiencing is actually not aware or attached the act. They simply begin to become that which they are experiencing. Finally, *Samadhi* is the experience of true union beyond the consciousness that we know in our physical and mental faculties. In this state, the ego and our attachments to the world no longer exist. This is the goal of the Eight-Limbed Path of Yoga.

Tristhana Method

The Tristhana Method refers to the combination of three essential elements in a yoga practice. They are the breath, the body posture, and the focus of the eyes. In Sanskrit, the eye focus is called the *dristhi*. These three things are practiced simultaneously during each posture to cleanse the body, mind, and nervous system.

Bandhas

The **bandhas** are energetic locks in the body. There are three basic areas where they are activated. **Mula** bandha is located at the bottom of the pelvic floor and is called the root lock. Try to gently lift the area between your sitting bones and pubic inward and upward to activate mula bandha. **Uddiyana** bandha is located just below the navel and translates to "flying up". To activate this bandha, lift your abdominal wall inward to the spine and upward toward the rib cage with elasticity. Do not harden the abdominal muscles- think of it as an internal lift. **Jalandhara** bandha is located at the throat and helps to control the flow of energy in your neck. To practice this lock, pull your chin back and then tuck it down to the chest.

Many of these bandhas are incorporated into yoga postures and pranayama techniques.

There are many popular styles of hatha yoga that are largely based around the practice of asana. They are listed as follows:

1. **Vinyasa/Flow:** a flowing style of yoga connecting several postures together, or practicing the Sun Salutation as a connective "vinyasa" between sequences of postures
2. **Ashtanga:** The basis of all vinyasa styles practiced today, it is a vigorous, regimented series of postures practiced in a set sequence utilizing vinyasa between every pose. Founded by Sri K. Pattahbi Jois.
3. **Iyengar:** a more static version of hatha yoga that utilizes long holds of postures and the use of props without any vinyasa. Focuses on alignment. Created by B.K.S. Iyengar
4. **Anusara:** blend of alignment based, flow, and Tantra philosophy. Designed by John Friend.

5. **Hot Yoga**: yoga that is practiced in a room heated to 100-105 degrees with up to 40% humidity. Originally conceived by Bikram Choudhury to include a set sequence, however many now practice vinyasa in heated rooms. It is said to promote detoxification in the body and increase flexibility.

6. **Kundalini:** Utilizes the postures with movement and breathing techniques to awaken dormant energy in the spine. Often the breath is cleansing, quick, and powerful.

7. **Restorative:** A gentle form of yoga that consists of postures performed mostly seated or reclined, often with the use of props for support. Poses are held for longer amounts of time to promote relaxation. Great for the elderly or those with injuries.

8. **Yin Yoga:** A slow and gentle style of yoga with long holds of postures

How to Start Practicing Yoga

To begin practicing yoga, you will need:

1. A yoga mat
2. 1 or 2 yoga blocks
3. A yoga strap or belt
4. A blanket
5. Comfortable, form fitting clothing
6. A quiet space free of distraction

You can find quality yoga mats at most sporting good or large retail stores. They may also carry the additional props as well. It is recommend using these extra props, especially in the beginning, because they will help you modify poses. Many postures may need the use of these props in the beginning to help you achieve the right alignment and support. Blocks are commonly used under the hands in forward bends or lunging positions, while straps can be used to connect our hands to body parts which may otherwise be inaccessible. They are very helpful for beginners.

Wearing comfortable clothing is also advisable when practicing yoga. When practicing hatha yoga in particular, you will want to wear more form fitting clothing that will not interfere with your movements or restrict your body in any way.

A quiet space free of distraction is equally important when practicing yoga, especially in the beginning. This will help to focus the mind on what you are doing, and allow you to cultivate a space for inner contemplation. Your space does not need to be large, but should have enough for your mat to fit and for you to be able to extend your arms out in any direction without being obstructed. You can decorate the space with objects that invoke particular meaning for you if you like. You could practice in your kitchen, living room, or backyard.

Centering

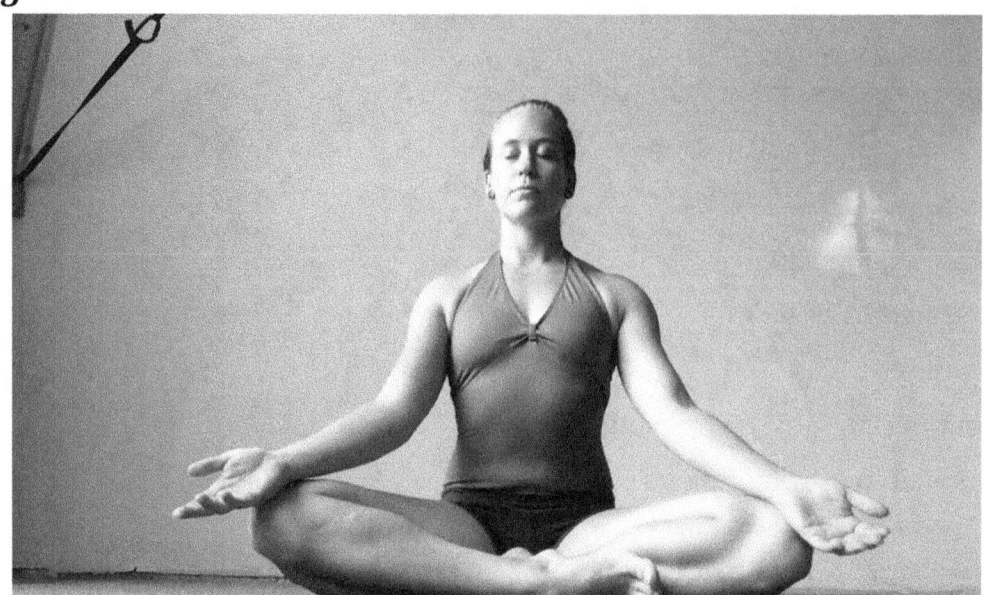

Once you feel that you have everything you need to begin practicing yoga, you are ready to start. Set up your mat and props in your yoga practice area. Take your shoes off and turn off your cell phone. Depending on the style of yoga you are practicing, you can begin seated, reclined, or standing. Close your eyes and bring your attention to your breath. Allow any lingering thoughts to drift away. Connecting to the breath will clear your mind and bring you into the present moment. Release any tensions, stresses, or worries through the body and the mind in this opening practice. One of the greatest lessons we can learn to inhabit is learning to be in the present moment with yourself.

If you find it difficult to clear your mind, try not to force it. The thoughts are not going to disappear automatically or in one sitting. Be patient with yourself. There are many techniques you can use to center yourself.

Breathe in and out through your nose when you begin to sit quietly. Lengthen your inhalation and exhalation until they are even in length. Take as many or as few breaths as you feel necessary in the beginning. Try to keep this balanced, deep breath in and out through the nose for the duration of your practice. Never inhale through your mouth.

Starting Seated

Starting your yoga practice in a comfortable seated position is a great way to begin. There are many ways you can choose to sit. The most common is to assume *Sukhasana*, or Easy Pose. In this position, you sit with your legs crossed. If this is not comfortable for you, it is recommended to first try sitting on a block or a folded blanket. If you have any hip or knee injuries, you can try sitting with your legs extended straight out in front of you. When seated, try to sit with a nice, long spine. Stack your shoulders right over your hips and feel your chest broad and open. Relax your shoulders away from your ears and lengthen the crown of your head toward the sky. Feel your tailbone rooting down into the earth. Connecting to your alignment and breath at the beginning of your practice will help to set the tone for the duration of your practice. Try to relax your hips and legs.

Starting Reclined

Lying down on your back is another way you can begin your practice. You can lay in *Savasana*, or Corpse Pose, with your legs extended out to the corner edges of your mat and your arms down by your sides with the palms face up. Or, you can start with your legs bent and your feet on the mat. If you are going to start on your back, allow yourself to relax with awareness of your body and breath. Feel your shoulders and hips pressing into the floor, and your spine nice and long in the center of your body. Allow your back to relax into the floor.

3 Part Breath

There is an easy way to connect to your breath when lying on your back. This type of breathing is called a 3 Part Breath, and is outlined here:

1. Take one hand and place it on your belly
2. Begin to feel your breath physically inside your body; sense the rise and fall of your belly with your breath. Feel your hand moving up and down as you inhale and exhale.
3. Place your other hand over your rib cage.
4. Now feel your belly and your rib cage fill with air as your inhale, and deflate completely as you exhale.
5. Continue this breathing for at least 5 breaths
6. Then, take your bottom hand and place it over the center of your chest
7. Feel your abdomen, rib cage, and chest expand as you inhale, and then send the breath all the way back down as you exhale.
8. Continue your 3 Part Breath for 5-10 breaths, or as many as you like.

The 3 Part Breath is a great way to understand how to deepen your breath and use your full lung capacity during your practice.

Starting Standing

Some yoga practices, such as the Ashtanga method, will begin standing in *Tadasana*, or Mountain Pose. In this basic standing posture, bring your feet directly under hips. The traditional variation of this pose calls for the big toes to come together with the heels slightly apart to promote a slight internal rotation of the legs. However, if this is uncomfortable at first, you can begin in a more open parallel position. The open parallel position is great because it will help to correct alignment issues in the legs and hips, and mirrors the way we should walk in our daily lives. Make sure that your toes, heels, knees, and hips are lined up in a straight line. For either variation, you also want to feel your shoulders stacked over the hips, and the hips stacked over the heels. Allow the spine to lengthen, the abdominals to gently draw inward, and the tailbone to lengthen downward.

Starting a yoga practice by standing is a good way to energize the body for a more active yoga practice you may be engaging in. However, it is slightly less meditative than the other methods of beginning and may be more difficult to connect to the breath. It is recommended to try the other methods first before trying this one.

Child's Pose

Child's Pose is one of the most foundational yoga postures to know. You can start in this posture and come back to it at any time. To try this one, come on to your hands and knees. Press your hips back to your heels and allow your brow to rest on the floor. Stretch your arms forward, or lay them alongside your hips.

If your head does not reach the floor, place a block under your forehead. If your hips do not reach your heels, you can roll up a blanket and place it between your hips and your heels. If you have sensitive knees when kneeling, you can either try to double up your mat or place a blanket under your knees.

Childs Pose, or *Balasana*, in Sanskrit, is a great way to release the muscles in the hips, lower back, and shoulders. It is overall a very relaxing and restorative posture both physically and energetically. It is a great way to begin a practice because it is easy to connect to the breath in the front and back side of the body. You can feel the rise and fall of the belly with the breath with ease in this position. You can also feel the lower back, back of the ribs, and back of the shoulders expand and condense as you inhale and exhale. This is also a great position to come back to if you ever feel overtaxed physically or disconnected to your breath when you are practicing.

Warming Up

Once you feel centered, it is important to begin with some easy warm up exercises and stretches. These movements and postures will help to activate the breath and body through movement and wake up the spine.

Breathing Up and Down

1. Sit in Easy Pose
2. Inhale and raise your hands up to the sky
3. Exhale and lower the arms back down toward the earth
4. Try to match your inhalation to the peak of your movements up and down
5. Allow your movements and breath to be slow and steady
6. Repeat at least 4 times.

Continuing from a seated position, there are a few options you can perform. A great way to open the back and the hips gently is to simply fold forward with your legs in the easy crossed position. Continue to breathe into the belly and the back, and relax the jaw. Then, you roll yourself up through your spine one vertebrae at a time. From there, take a twist over your right shoulder by reaching your left hand to your right knee and your right hand behind you. Do not force anything in this twist, just feel the gentle rotation of the spine lifting inward and upward. Take 3-5 breaths in each stretch. After the first side, notice which leg you have crossed in front, and change sides so the other leg is in front. Repeat on the other side.

You can also stretch your neck from side to side while seated.

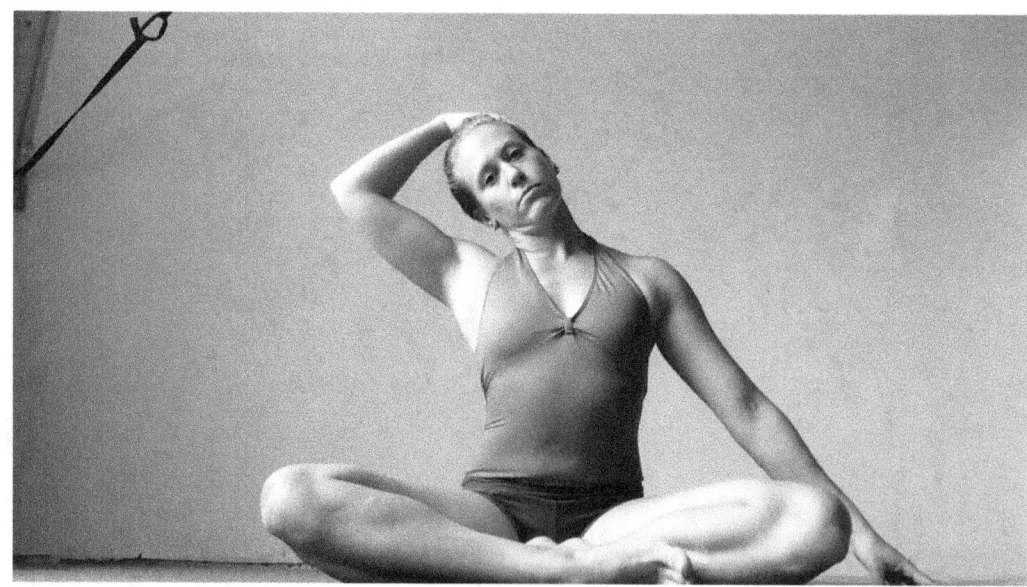

Basic Postures

Cat/Cow

Come onto your hands and knees, establishing a tabletop position. Stack your shoulders over your wrists and your hips over your knees. Toes can be tucked under or untucked. Lengthen the spine and feel the crown of the head stretching forward. Lift the belly muscles upward away from the mat. Spread through all ten fingers, and draw the shoulders into the back, away from the ears. Take a few breaths here to center and find your alignment.

Once you have your foundation established, you can begin what is called Cat/Cow. This is a great exercise to wake up the spine and get it moving in a healthy way. It combines two stretches into an easy sequence.

1. On an exhalation, round your back like a cat. Curl your head and tail under and make a C-curve with your spine.
2. On an inhalation, reverse the curve of your spine so that you are arching your back and dropping your belly downward. Curve your head and tail upward while also looking upward.
3. Continue rolling through the spine up and down feeling the fluidity of its movement
4. Allow each movement and breath to be synced up and expansive
5. Repeat each set at least 5 times

This activity is great for getting the circulation moving through your body. It should feel like a gentle flowing movement in the body. It will also improve your balance, strengthen and stretch the muscles of the back, abdomen, and hips, as well as increase your coordination, and relieve stress.

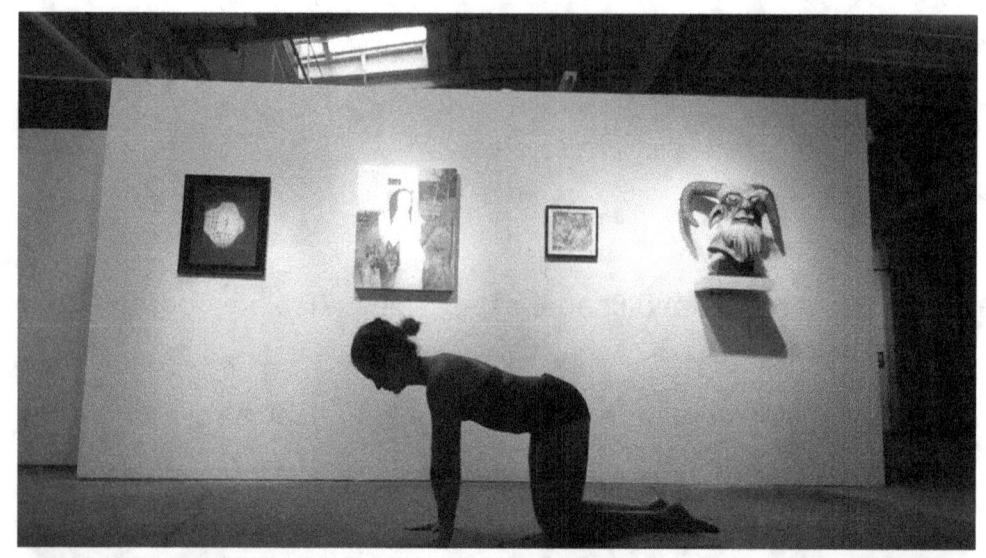

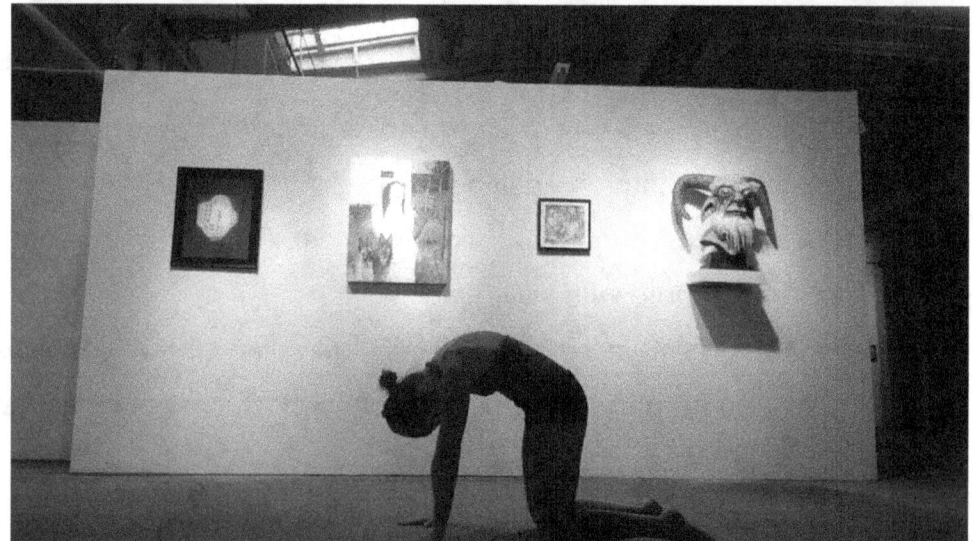

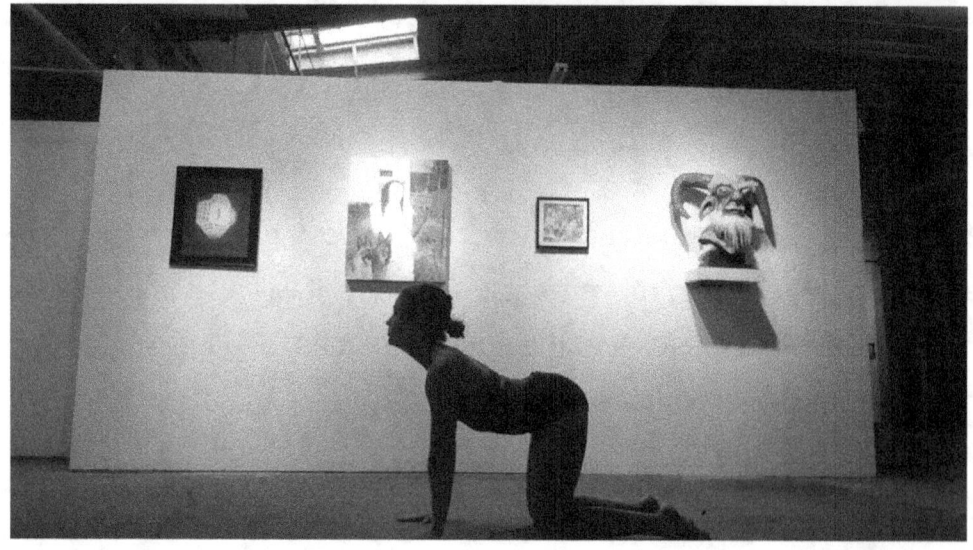

Downward Facing Dog (Adho Mukha Svanasana)

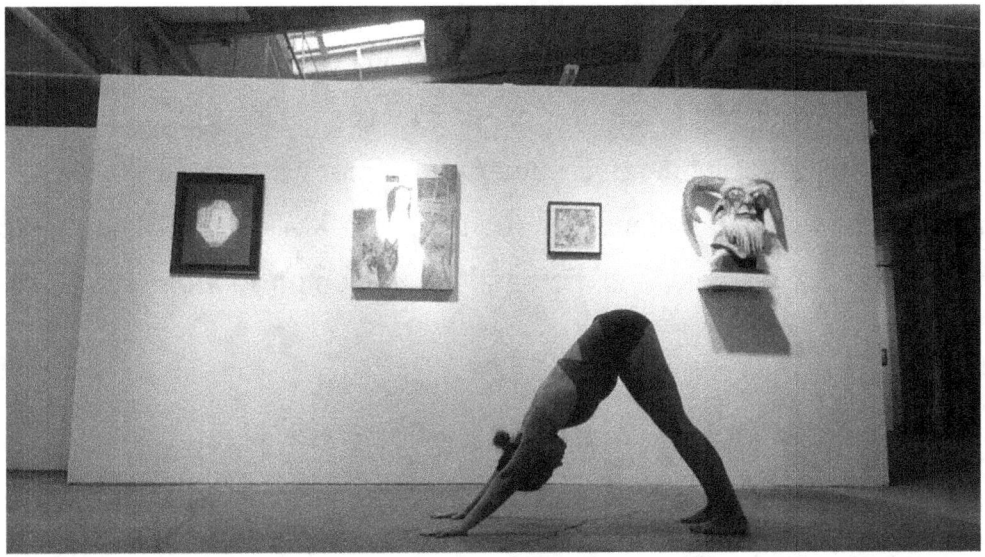

Establish your foundation in tabletop position. Then, begin to move into Downward Dog by following these steps:

1. Tuck your toes under
2. Lift your hips so that your body makes an inverted V-shape
3. Press your heels toward the floor
4. Lengthen the spine
5. Press the chest through the arms
6. Draw the shoulders away from the ears and relax the neck
7. Lengthen the legs as much as possible
8. Keep your feet in a nice parallel position in line with the hips

If you find it difficult to lengthen your legs or your back in Downward Facing Dog, modify by stepping your feet an inch closer to your hands. Then, keep your knees slightly bent to work on lengthening the spine. Once the spine can fully extend in this position, you will be ready to work on straightening out the legs. It does not have to happen right away, so give yourself plenty of time. This yoga posture is a timeless one because it is done in almost every practice several times, depending on the style.

The benefits of Downward Dog are vast. It will strengthen your hands and wrists, as well as stretch your back, hamstrings, and calves. This stretching and strengthening posture will help decrease pain in your back and shoulders. It is also known to help relieve tension and headaches by naturally elongating the spine and relaxing the head. It also helps to increase circulation throughout your entire body.

Cobra (Bhujangasana)

Cobra is a wonderful spine strengthening posture. To begin, follow these steps:

1. Lay on the front surface of your body, belly down to the floor

2. Line up your feet with your hips; toes are pointed

3. Place your hands as close to under your shoulders as you can. Your elbows will lift off the ground in this position.

4. Tuck your elbows into the sides of your body, activating your triceps.

5. Keeping your elbows tucked in and your neck nice and long, begin to lift a few inches off of the mat.

6. Press down into the hands and lift a little higher, beginning to stretch the abdomen. Draw the belly muscles in away from the floor so they are active and to protect the lower back in this position.

7. Make sure your arms are not doing all of the work; try to lift from your back.

8. Eventually your arms can straighten, but they do not have to.

If you feel like you are straining or have a back injury, you can modify with a Sphinx pose. In Sphinx, you will place your elbows right under your shoulders instead of your hands. Line up your wrists with your elbows and press your forearms into the mat while lifting your chest and extending your spine upwards. Maintain similar muscular action and alignment principals of the Cobra to receive the maximum benefits.

The benefits of cobra pose include decreased back stiffness, increased back and arm strength, an elevated mood, and improved digestion.

Plank Pose

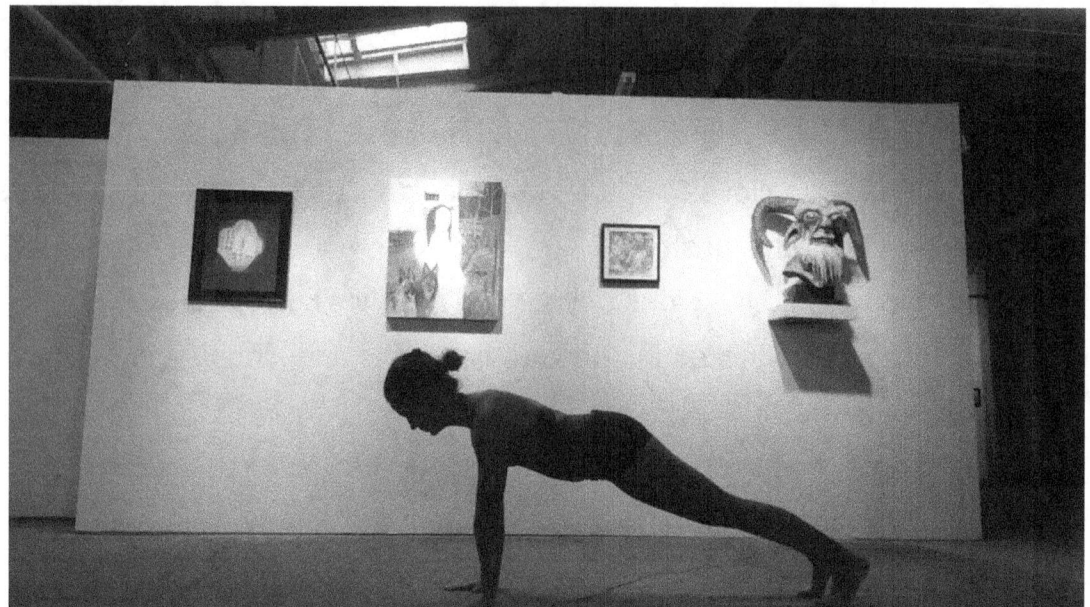

Plank Pose is a foundational strength posture. To perform this posture, follow these steps:

1. Set up your tabletop position
2. Extend one foot at a time behind you with your toes tucked under and heels pressing backward
3. Keep your body in a straight line without hanging in the hips or the head
4. Engage your abdominals by drawing them upward and connecting your rib cage inward
5. Keep the shoulders stacked directly over the wrists
6. Feel the shoulder blades moving gently in toward the center of your body
7. Make sure the hips are not elevated

This posture can be especially challenging in the beginning. If your strength is not quite there to hold this position yet or you have any injuries that prevent you from performing this, you can try the modified variation. To modify, drop the knees to the mat (but not the hips). Keep all of the other alignment cues in mind. Make sure you are not in a tabletop position. In modified plank, the knees will be slightly behind the hips, creating a downward sloping diagonal line.

Plank pose is a whole body strengthener. It will help to improve posture by strengthening the shoulder girdle and abdominals. It is also a great exercise in willpower and will increase your mental capacity to perform well under pressure.

Standing Forward Fold (Uttanasana)

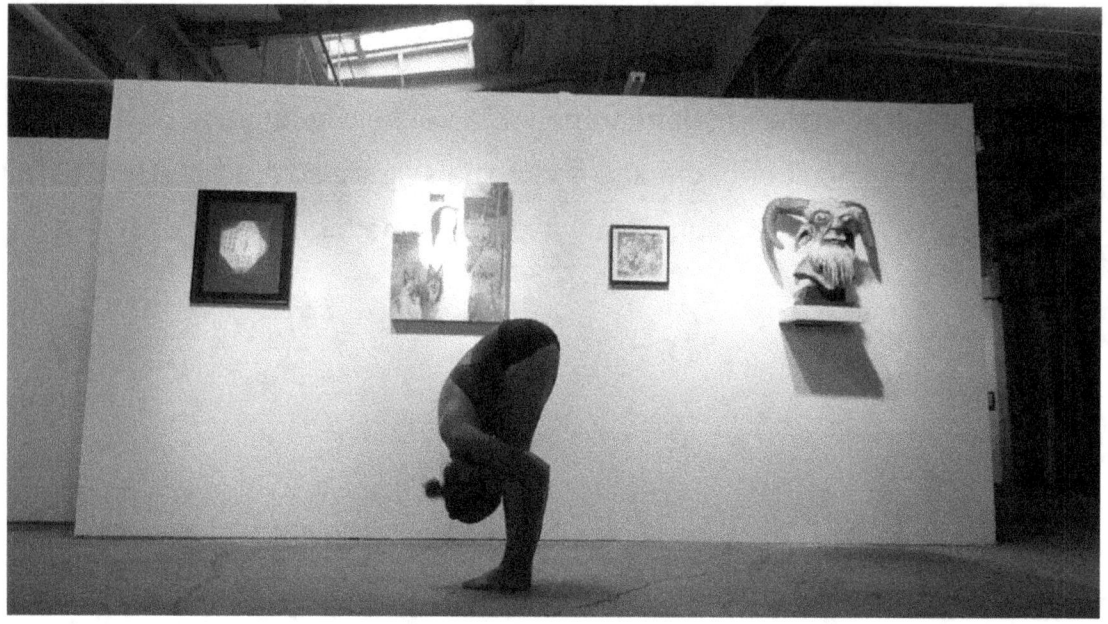

Uttanasana is a standing forward fold that stretches the back and hamstrings. Start in Mountain Pose. On an exhale begin to fold forward by creasing at the hips. Use a block under your hands or hold onto your shins if your hands do not reach the floor. Or, clasp onto the calves to deepen the stretch for more flexibility. It is okay if the knees are slightly bent. Make sure your body weight is toward the toes to prevent the knees from locking. This pose can be performed in either the narrow or more open parallel position of the feet.

Variations

To stretch the shoulders in a forward fold, clasp the hands behind the back while in Mountain Pose. Fold forward, taking your hands up behind you as you fold. If your shoulders are tight, try holding onto a strap with your hands a little further apart.

For a restorative variation, try hanging in the forward fold like a rag doll. Soften your knees and back while holding on to opposite elbows. Take a gentle sway from side to side through your torso, or gently rock your head to release the neck muscles. Feel as if water could gently cascade off of your back.

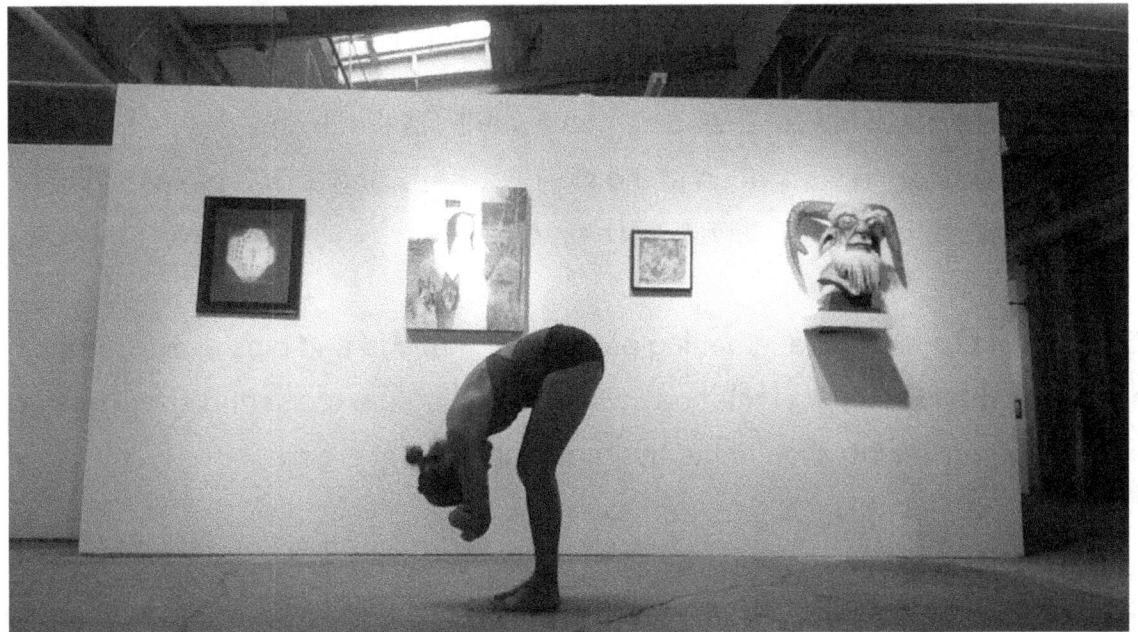

Chair Pose (Utkatasana)

Utkatasana translates to the "pose of fierceness" and if often referred to as chair pose. The reason for its ferocity is because it activates the quadriceps intensely. To perform this posture, follow these steps:

1. Stand in Mountain Pose in either the narrow parallel or open parallel position
2. Bend your knees
3. Line up your knees directly with your toes
4. Shift the weight of your body slightly toward your heels so that you can lift your toes lightly off the floor
5. Squeeze your inner thighs together if your big toes are touching in the narrow version
6. Curl the tailbone slightly under
7. Scoop the navel toward the spine and away from the thighs
8. Reach your arms straight up to the sky. You can connect the palms together if that is comfortable but it is not necessary.

Chair pose is a great strengthening posture for the legs and hips. It encourages stability in the lower half of the body while stretching the chest and shoulders. It will also encourage stimulation of the heart and abdominal organs.

Warrior 1 (Virabhadrasana I)

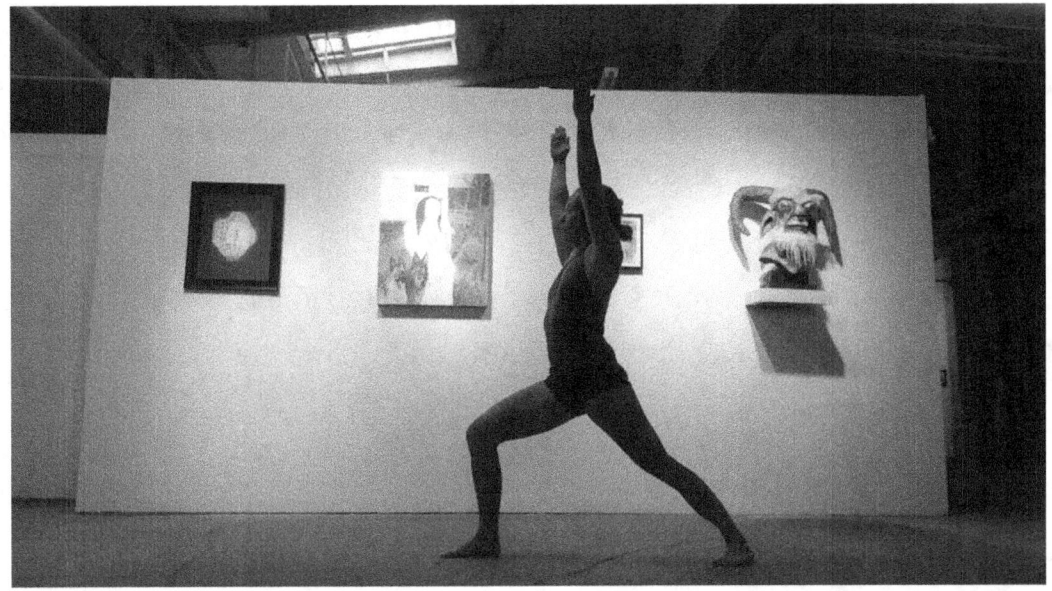

Warrior 1 is another foundational yoga posture that you can practice regularly. To perform this posture, step one foot back from Mountain Pose. Turn the back foot out about 45 degrees, so that it is pointed slightly forward on diagonal. Try to press your heel down into the floor. Bend your front knee and straighten the back leg. Keep your front knee stacked over your ankle. Reach your arms up to the sky. You can connect your palms if you want, but it is not necessary in the beginning. Try to keep your hips pointing forward as much as possible. To accomplish this, pull the hip bone of your front leg back and spiral the hip bone of your back leg forward. Relax your shoulders away from your ears so your neck is nice and long.

Warrior 1 is a posture of strength, bravery, and graciousness. It stretches the hips, calves, and shoulders. It also connects your feet to the earth and lifts your heart to the sky, creating an energetic balance in the body of equality.

Crescent Side Stretch Pose

Side Crescent is another great warm up posture. It stretches the side body while increasing your lung capacity. From your basic standing position, reach your left arm up to the sky and then lean over to the right side. You want to feel this as an arch through the body. Keep your right arm pressed into the right side of your body and drag your finger tips down the leg to create extra space for the stretch to the grow. Think of rolling your top shoulder back so that your shoulders are stacked in a line. Keep your eyes forward so that your head does not drop. Breathe deeply into the lungs, increasing the space between your ribs.

High Lunge

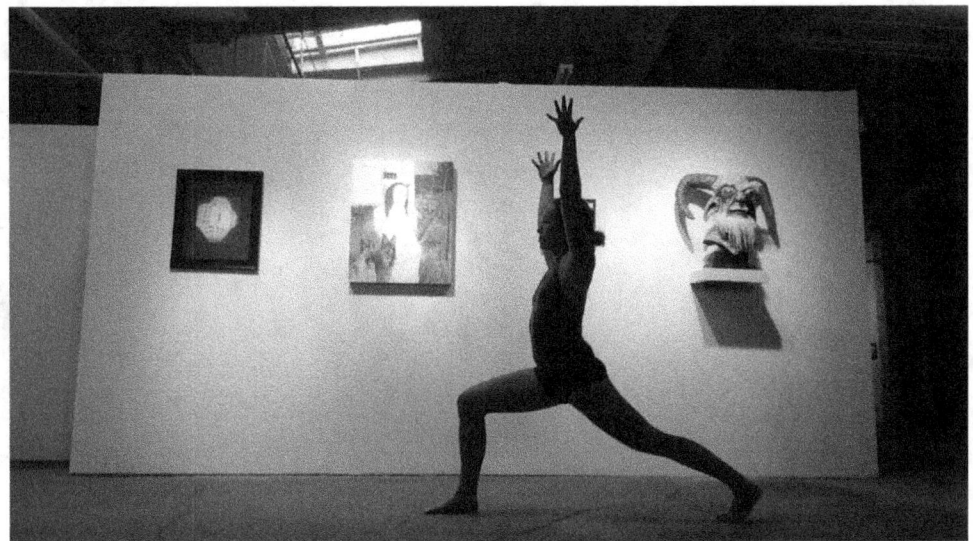

High Lunge is a fantastic hip opener and leg strengthener. It is also a great way to modify Warrior 1 if you have trouble keeping the back heel down. To move into this posture, start in a forward fold. With your hands on the floor, step your left leg as far back as you can behind you. Keep your toes tucked under with your lifted and pressing toward the back edge of your mat. Make sure that your front knee stays stacked over your ankle, making a 90 degree angle with your leg. Place your hands on either of your front foot.

If you have difficulty achieving this, place two blocks on either side of your front foot. This little bit of elevation will allow your torso to come slightly, creating space for your body to align itself properly. You can also try wiggling your back foot a bit further back after that first step to increase the stretch. You can also modify by bringing the back knee down to the mat.

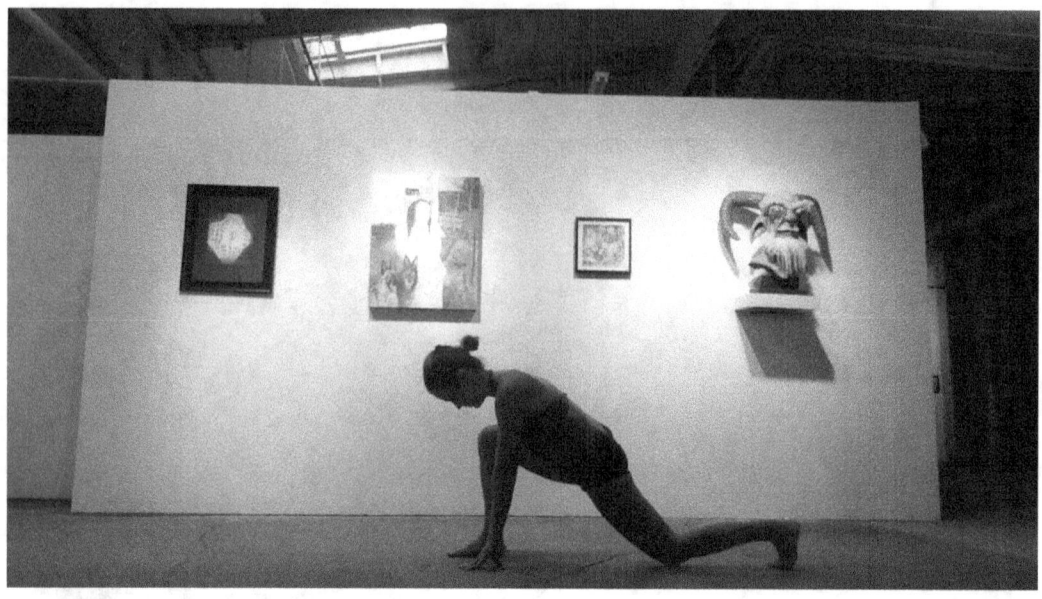

To increase the stretch or challenge your strength, try taking your hands onto your front thigh. You can also try to balance by extending your arms all the way up to the sky.

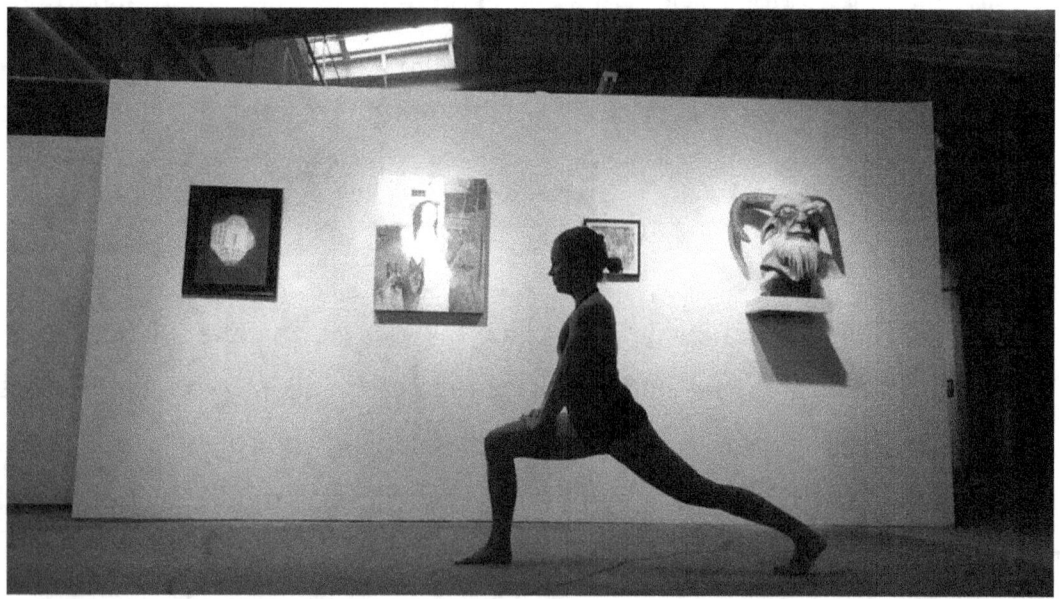

This will stretch the hip flexors deeply and open the front side of the body.

Revolved Lunge

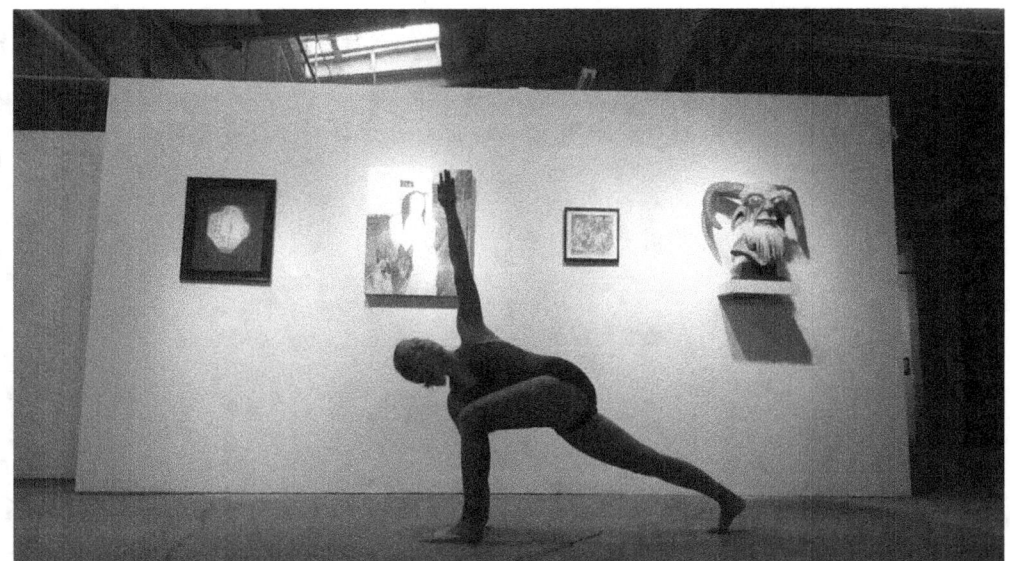

From your basic lunging position you can take an easy twist. Twists are great cleansing actions for the inner body. Twists also help to relieve back pain and tone the abdominals. Traditionally, you always want to twist to the right side first. This is because this action massages the ascending colon and promotes good digestion.

To perform this easy twist, place your left hand under shoulder while in a high or low lunge (knee down to the floor). Extend your right arm straight up to the sky, keeping the shoulder blades engaged into the back. Spiral your belly muscles away from the front thigh. Imagine that you are wringing out your core like a wet sponge.

Warrior 2 (Virabhadrasana II)

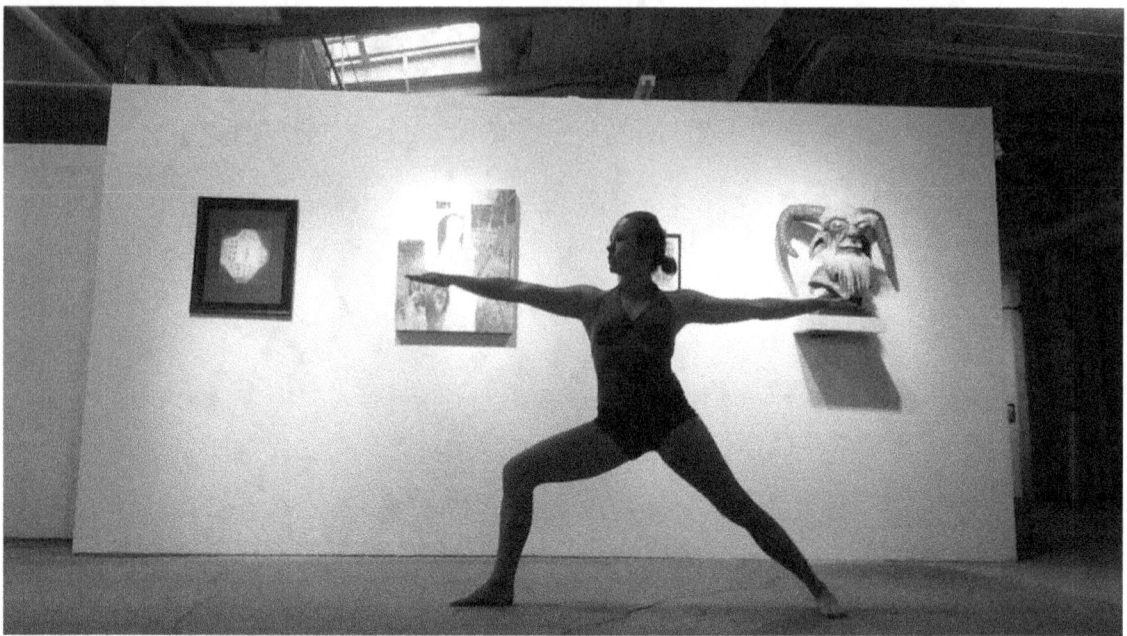

Warrior 2 (*Virabhadrasana II*) is another foundational yoga posture. It opens the hips by grounding the feet and legs toward the earth. Keep one foot pointing forward and step your other foot way back. Turn the back foot and the entire torso out to the side. Bend the front knee and lengthen the back leg. Sink the hips down. Relax the shoulders and focus the eyes over the front hand. This is a great posture to focus the gaze and feel the steadiness of a single pointed focus. To find success whether doing yoga or anything else in life, a steady and focused mind is essential. Hold for 3-5 breaths.

The benefits of Warrior 2 include toned leg muscles and an increased sense of energy. It will improve your sense of concentration in your mind as well. It will also help improve your circulation throughout your entire body.

Extended Side Angle Pose (Parsvakonasana)

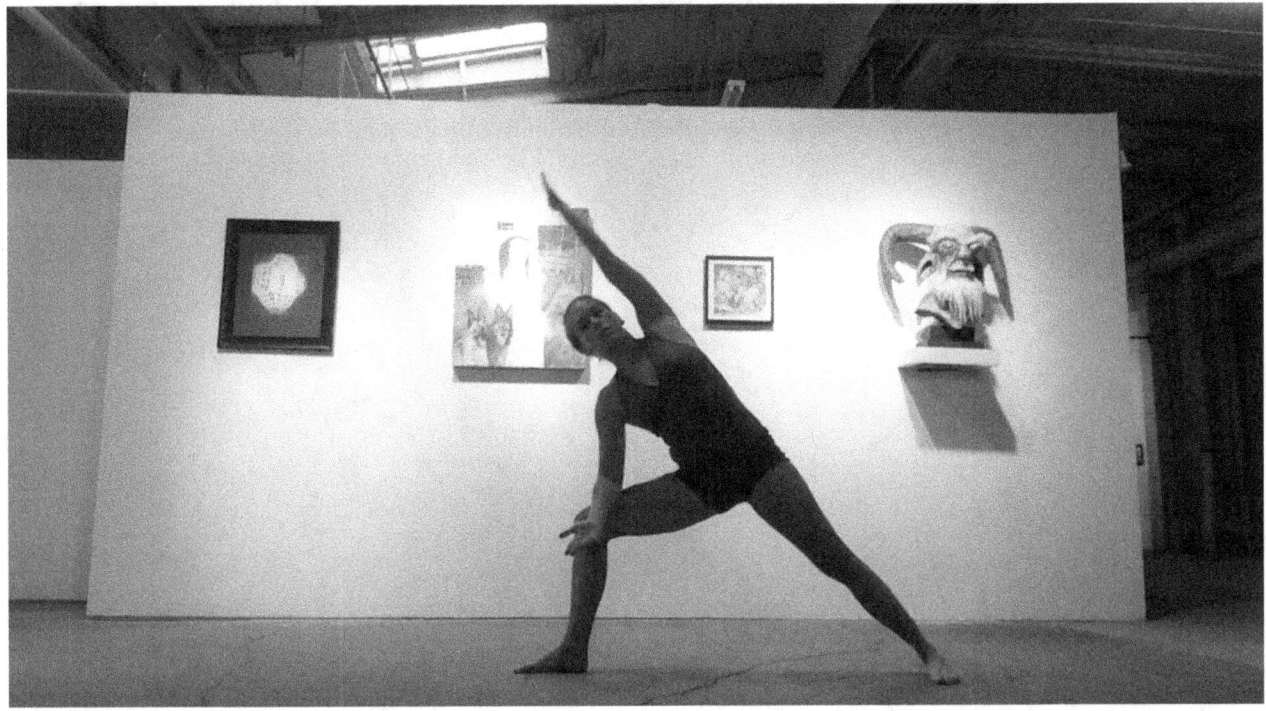

Keep your legs in the same position as Warrior 2 and move your torso diagonally over the front bent leg, standing the same arm as leg on the thigh. Take the opposite arm and reach it as far forward by the ear as you can. Continue pressing through the outer edge of your back leg and drawing the core in. Feel the side stretch on the open side of the body from under the shoulder all the way down to the hip. This wonderful side stretch is essential to opening up those muscles under the shoulder blade. Feel your lungs expand fully as you inhale and exhale.

To modify this posture for tight shoulders, take your top extended arm and place your hand behind your head. Your arm will be bent in this modified position. Feel your elbow lifting up and back into the side plane of your body. To deepen the pose, try to reach your bottom arm to the inside or outside of your front foot. It is okay if you cannot reach the floor. You can stack a block underneath of your hand for support.

Side Angle is a great posture that can help to relieve stiffness in the neck and shoulders while also stretching the hips. It continues to encourage a sense of groundedness through the legs as well. Side angle will also tone the abdominals and help to ease pain from sciatica.

Triangle Pose (Trikonasana)

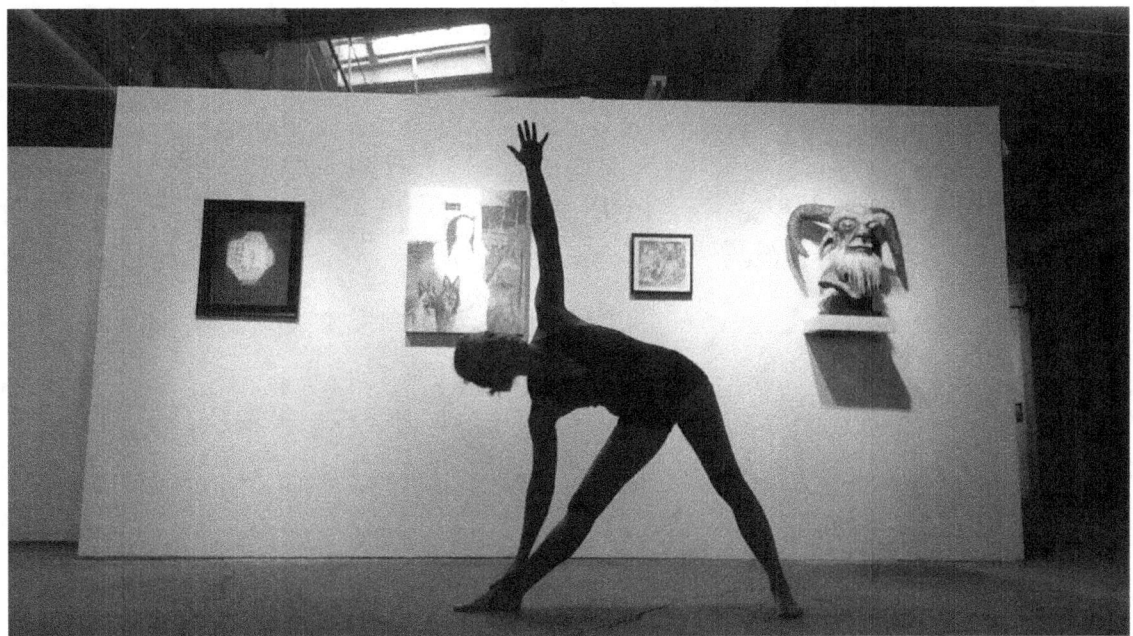

To perform Triangle Pose, follow these guidelines:

1. From Mountain Pose, step your left back and turn it out to face the side.
2. Face your entire torso to the same side and raise your arms to a T-shape in line with your shoulders.
3. Reach as far over the right leg as you can, keeping your shoulders in line with your front leg.
4. Place your bottom hand on your shin or ankle. You can also place it on a block in front of or behind the front leg for support.
5. Continue reaching your top arm and hand upward to the sky, creating a straight line with the arms.
6. Root down through your feet and feel the muscles of your legs spiraling inward and upward.
7. Pull your kneecaps upward and do not lock your knees. If they do tend to lock, keep them at a soft bend.
8. To move out of the pose, come back up to standing on an inhalation.

Pyramid Pose (Parsvottanasana)

Pyramid Pose is a great posture that lengthens the hamstrings and back while promoting balance in the body. To perform this posture, step your left food back from Mountain Pose. Turn your back foot out slightly while keeping your hips square to the front of your mat. To keep your hips square, you will want to feel a straight line across your hip bones. If they feel uneven, you can pull your hip bone back while pressing the left hip bone forward.

Once your foundation is established, you can fold forward into a more full extension of the posture. Place your hands on either side of your front foot. If they do not reach, you can either hold on to your shin or place a block under either hand for support. To come out of the posture, lift back up to standing while inhaling.

Standing Wide Legged Forward Fold (Prasarita Padottanasana)

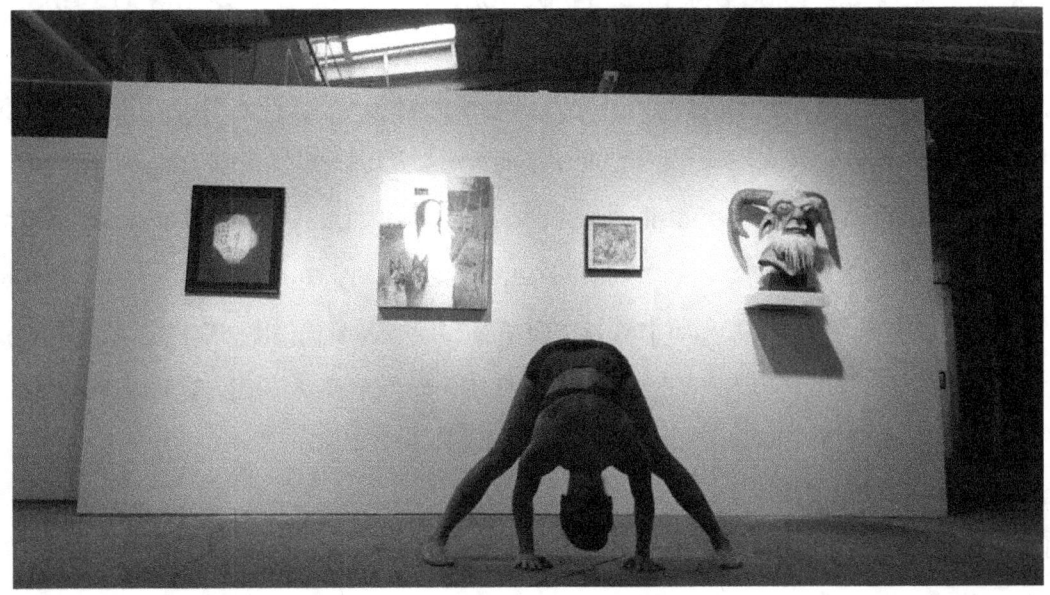

How to do Wide Legged Forward Fold:

1. Step out to the side and extend your arms to a T position
2. Line up your ankles underneath of your wrists and point your toes forward in a parallel position as if you were standing on wide railroad tracks
3. Inhale to lengthen the spine
4. Exhale and hinge forward at the hips.
5. You can place the hands on the mat or on a block if they do not reach the floor.
6. Try to lengthen your spine by drawing the shoulders away from the floor and toward your hips
7. Make sure the weight is toward the toes so the knees are not locked
8. It is okay if you need to bend your knees in this position.

Standing Leg Extension (*Uttitha Hasta Padangustasana*)

This posture is a standing balance. To perform this pose, follow these steps:

1. Standing on both feet evenly, lift up all ten toes and spread them back down into the mat from your pinky toes to your big toes. This will allow you to root down through your feet energetically to stimulate your ability to balance efficiently.
2. Place your hands on your hips and make sure they are even.
3. Keep your left hand on your left hip and shift your weight onto your left leg.
4. Pick up your right knee with your right hand and bend it into the chest.
5. After 3-5 breaths, move the right knee out to the side.
6. Stay here for another 3-5 breaths.
7. To come out of the posture, move the knee back forward and release to standing on both feet.
8. Repeat by picking up the left leg.

Advancing Standing Leg Extension

To advance this balancing posture, try this:

1. Instead of reaching for your knee in the balance, reach for your big toe instead and hold on tight.
2. Flexing your foot, begin to press your foot forward into your hand.
3. If your leg does not straighten, that is okay. You can keep your leg bent.
4. Keep your chest lifted and spine long- do not compromise by sinking your chest or rounding your shoulders

Modifications for Standing Leg Extension

1. If you are having trouble balancing, you can try to step off your mat and onto a harder surface for more stability.

2. Step over to a wall to stabilize your balance in this posture. If you are lifting the right knee, you will place your left hand on the wall. In this variation, you can "test" your balance by lightly taking your hand off the wall and then using it again when you need it, know that it is there for you.

Tree Pose (Vrksasana)

Tree Pose is one of the most well known and loved yoga postures. There are many variations and modifications you can take when first learning this pose. To start this balance, follow these guidelines:

1. Standing on your left foot, turn your right knee out to the side.
2. Place your right foot on your calf or above your knee to the top part of your inner thigh. Do not place the foot on your knee; this will compromise your balance if you do. If your foot will not reach any higher than your knee, practice the foot at a lower position until your hips are more open accommodate the higher position.
3. Place your hands at heart center.
4. Keep your torso facing forward; do not twist toward the open leg.
5. Steady your gaze on a single point.
6. Breathe deeply into the trunk of your body.
7. Continue rooting down through the standing foot and reaching the crown upward toward the sky
8. To exit the posture, turn the right knee forward and place the foot back down on the ground.

Staff Pose (Dandasana)

Staff Pose is a deceptively simple pose. For this posture, you will come to a seated position on your mat. Extend both of your legs out in front of you. Rock side to side to pull the flesh away from your sitting bones to feel them rooting down into the earth. Squeeze your legs together as tightly as you can, flexing your feet. Feel your inner thighs pressing into the center of your body. Place your hands right beside your hips and press your palms into the mat, spreading all ten fingers wide. On an exhalation, tuck your chin to your chest. This will activate jalandhara bandha. At the same time activate mula bandha and uddiyana bandha by lifting the pelvic floor muscles and scooping the abdominals inward and upward. Try to keep your shoulders stacked over your hips without rounding them forward. If your lower back starts to round or you cannot straighten your legs all the way, try elevating your hips by sitting on a black. This will create additional space in your hamstrings and lower back. Hold for 3-5 breaths.

Seated Forward Fold (Paschimottanasana)

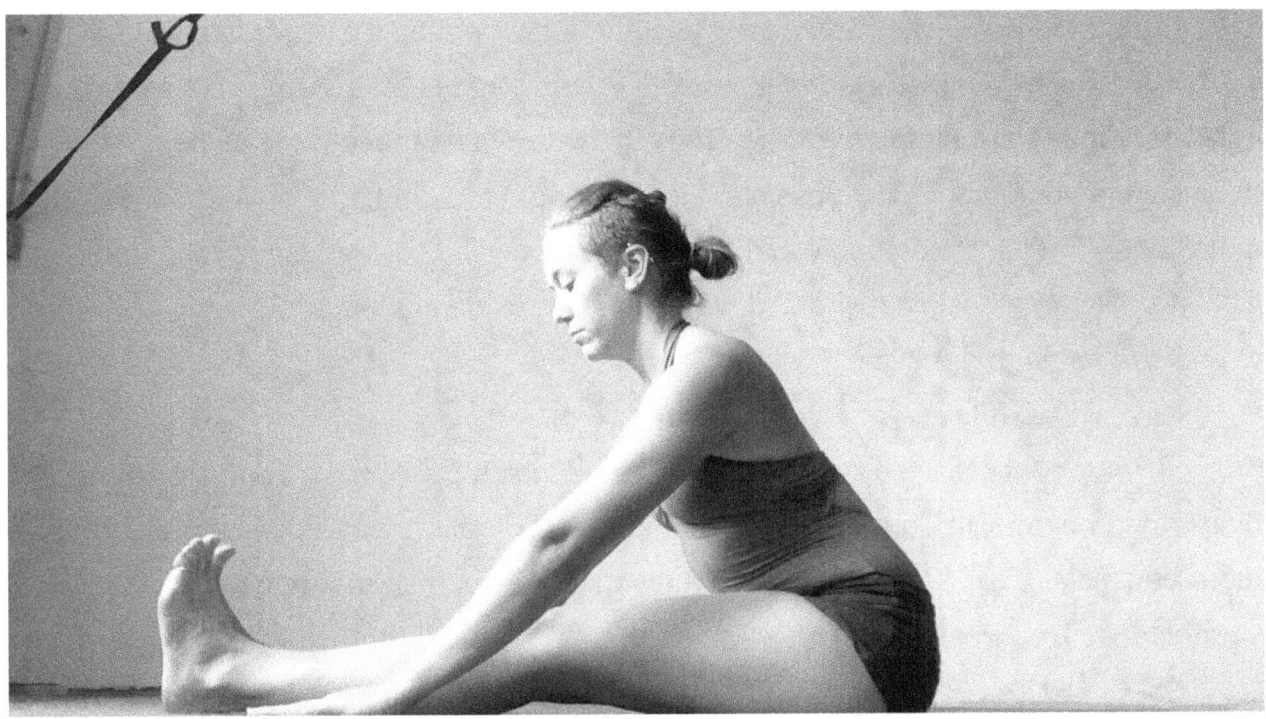

To take a seated forward fold, start with the legs in the same position as Staff Pose. Reach for your feet by folding forward at the hips. You can loop your pointer and middle finger around the big toe, or hold on to the outside of your feet. If you cannot reach your feet, you can either bend your legs as much as necessary or hold on to your shins. Other ways to modify include elevating your hips on a block, or looping a strap around your feet to hold on to.

One you are in the position, try to lengthen the neck by sliding the shoulders away from the ears. This will also help to elongate the upper back. Keep the belly muscles pulled in as well, so that you are not just collapsing over the legs. Keep the legs active by continually flexing the feet and pulling the toes back toward the hips. Hold for as many breaths as you would like.

Head to Knee Pose (Janu Sirsasana)

Head to Knee Pose is a forward fold and a hip opener. To move into this position, start seated with your legs extended straight out in front of you. Keep your right leg extended while bending the left knee out to the side. Place the left foot as high up on the inside of your right leg as possible. Flex your right foot and fold forward on an exhalation. You can hold on to either side of the foot with both hands, or your shin. Again, similar to a basic forward fold, you can also bend your leg and/or use your strap to find support in this position.

If your bent knee feels stiff or unsupported in this position, you can also place a block underneath of it. This will allow that hip to relax, soften, and open so the stretch is more beneficial. This is a great posture for working to improve the range of motion in your hips for Tree Pose.

While in the posture, try to lengthen your spine as much as possible. If your shoulders start to round at all, draw them into the back. Keep your abdominals engaged and breathe deeply.

Seated Twist

Performing seated twists are great ways to begin or end a yoga practice. They are calming postures that encourage gentle opening through the body. To practice this pose, start seated with both legs extended straight out in front of you. Bend your right knee into a half squat position, and step it over to the other side (across the left leg). Really feel as if you are standing on that right foot so that your foot firmly presses down.

Once your foundation is established, place your right hand directly behind you. On an inhalation, lift your left arm up. As you exhale, begin to twist through the center of your body toward the right knee. Cross your left arm over to the right side, bending the elbow and press it into the knee firmly. Keep the left fingertips spread and active. Look back over your right shoulder as far as you comfortably can.

In this twist, imagine that you are spiraling inward and upward from the base of the belly all the way up through the crown of the head. Pull the abdominals inward to tone the belly and protect the action of the spine. Do not force this twist. To modify for any tightness or injuries, do not hook the left elbow across the right knee. Instead, just simply hug the right knee. This will make the twist less impactful on the body.

Make sure to repeat on the other side.

Boat Pose (Navasana)

Boat Pose is one of the most well known abdominal strengthening positions. Follow these steps to perform this posture:

1. From seated, bend both knees and place your feet on the mat. Keep your legs squeezed together as tightly as you can, or keep them in line with your hips.
2. Grab underneath of your knees and begin to lean back.
3. Pick your feet up until your shins are parallel to the floor in a tabletop position
4. Lift your chest and relax your shoulders
5. Feel your abdominals scooping inward away from the thighs
6. Find your balance and breathe with steadiness
7. To test your balance, reach your arms straight out in front you
8. For an additional challenge, try to straighten your legs into a V-shape

Bridge Pose (Setu Bandhasana)

Bridge Pose is a great counter pose to perform after working the abdominals in boat pose. For this pose, lay all the way down on your back. Line up your heels with your sitting bones by bending the legs and keeping them in a parallel position. Place your arms right alongside the body. Begin to curl the tailbone under and peel the spine off of the mat one vertebrae at a time. This action will lift the hips up into the air. Press your arms firmly into the mat and engage your abdominals. Try to relax your neck.

To take this posture one step further, roll your shoulders underneath the body and clasp your hands together. This may lift your hips up a bit higher.

Begin to come out of the bridge by rolling back down through your spine sequentially one vertebrae at a time. Bend your knees into your chest, giving yourself a hug after this pose. Gently rock side to side to massage the lower back out.

Bridge pose is a great posture that stretches the front side of the body and massages the thyroid gland.

Bound Angle Pose (Baddha Konasana)

Bound angle pose is a great way to open your hips and stretch your back. From a seated position, bend both knees and place the soles of your feet together. Hold onto your ankles and sit tall. On an exhalation, begin to tuck the chin into the chest. Roll down through the spine, folding forward over the legs. You can stay here, keeping the head heavy, or walk the hands forward to increase the stretch in the hips. If your hips feel tight, place a block underneath each knee for support. Roll yourself back up gently to come out of the posture.

Eye of the Needle Pose (Sucirandhrasana)

Eye of the Needle Pose is a wonderful, easy hip opener. Lay all the way down on your back to start. Bend your legs so the feet come onto the mat. Cross your right ankle over your left. Thread your right hand through the center of both legs and grab above or below your left knee. Fold the legs into your chest and breathe into your right hip.

This posture will stretch your outer hips. This is a great stretch to use as a cool down posture. It is important to stretch this muscle group after performing poses such as high lunge and the Warriors, because the target the hip flexors on the inside of the hip.

If you have difficulty bending the legs into the chest or grabbing under the knee, you can assist yourself by using a strap. Loop the strap underneath of the leg you are grabbing. When you go to reach for that leg, hold onto your strap instead. This is a great way to modify if your outer hips are particularly tight.

Reclined Leg Extension

Lay down on your back to perform this posture and follow these steps:

1. Press your shoulders and hips into the mat evenly
2. Bend your right knee into your chest while rooting your left leg into the mat. If your hips are tight, bend your left leg and place the foot on the mat to modify.
3. Stay here for 3-5 breaths.
4. Keeping hold of your right knee, open it out to the side. Do not let your left hip come off of the mat. Hold for 3-5 breaths.
5. Return your knee to the center to exit.

To advance this stretch:

1. After bending the leg into the chest, hold onto the foot. If you cannot reach the foot, loop a strap around your foot.
2. Kick your foot upward to the sky, extending the leg as much as you can. It does not have to straighten all the way.
3. Take the leg out to the side, same as the first variation.
4. Bring the leg back to the center to finish.

Reclined Twist

A reclined twist is a great way to end your practice before Savasana. It is a very restorative posture and can help ease back pain. Lay down your back to move into this relaxing stretch. Then, fold both knees into your chest. Extend your arms to a T position. Let both legs release over to the right side. If it's comfortable, look over your left shoulder. Breathe into your hips, lower back, rib cage, and shoulders.

To come out of the posture, bring your legs back to the center and then repeat on the other side.

Corpse Pose (Savasana)

Savasana is one of the most important postures in yoga. It is performed at the very end of a practice or class. The title of the posture as Corpse Pose refers to this posture's ability to transform the yoga practitioner. It is a quiet place where we can experience our true nature fully.

To practice Savasana, extend your legs out to the corner edges of the mat and relax your legs. Extend your arms down by your side with your palms face upward. Lengthen your neck and relax your jaw. Close your eyes. Allow your breath to return to its natural state. Practice conscious awareness. This is not a place to simply fall asleep, but rather a place to become aware of the fruits of our practice. Stay here for 5 minutes or longer.

When you are ready to move out of Savasana, begin to deepen your breath. Gently move your fingers and toes to wake the body back up. Bend your knees into your chest and rock over to the right side. It is recommended to always rock over to the right side to promote blood flow from the heart. When you are ready, press yourself up to a comfortable seated position with ease.

Sun Salutations

Sun Salutation A (Surya Namaskar A)

A foundational sequence to warm up the whole body is the Sun Salutation A (*Surya Namaskar A*). Each movement is connected to the breath in this sequence. This forms the basis of the *vinyasa*, or flow, style of yoga. Here is a breakdown of the Sun Salutation A with some modifications:

1. Stand in Mountain Pose
2. Inhale and raise your arms overhead.

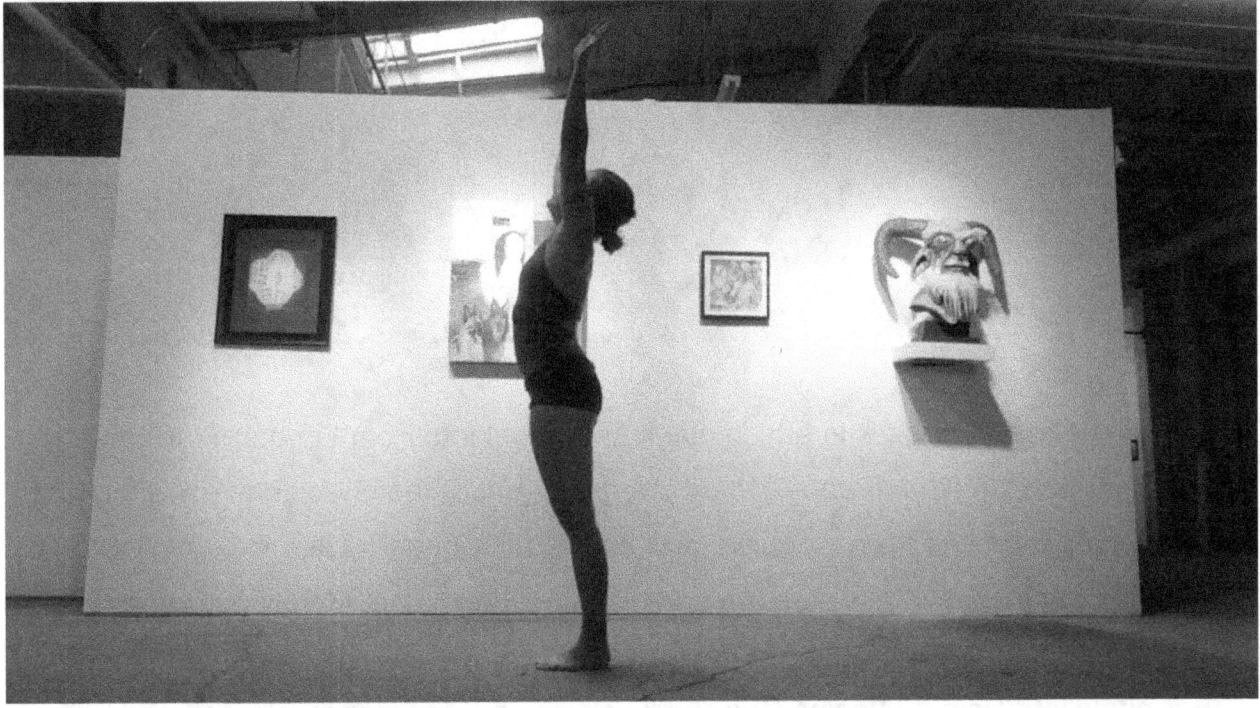

3. Exhale and fold forward completely. Hold onto your shins if your hands do not reach the floor. Or, clasp onto the calves to deepen the stretch for more flexibility. It is okay if the knees are slightly bent. Make sure your body weight is toward the toes to prevent the knees from locking.
4. Inhale to lengthen the spine and draw the shoulders away from the ears. You can lift up as high as you need to. In the beginning, it may be necessary to lift to a 90

degree angle so that your torso is parallel to the floor. If you have the mobility, you can keep your fingertips on the floor while you lift. Otherwise, keep them on your shins. Make sure you do not lock the knees; it is fine to bend them slightly.

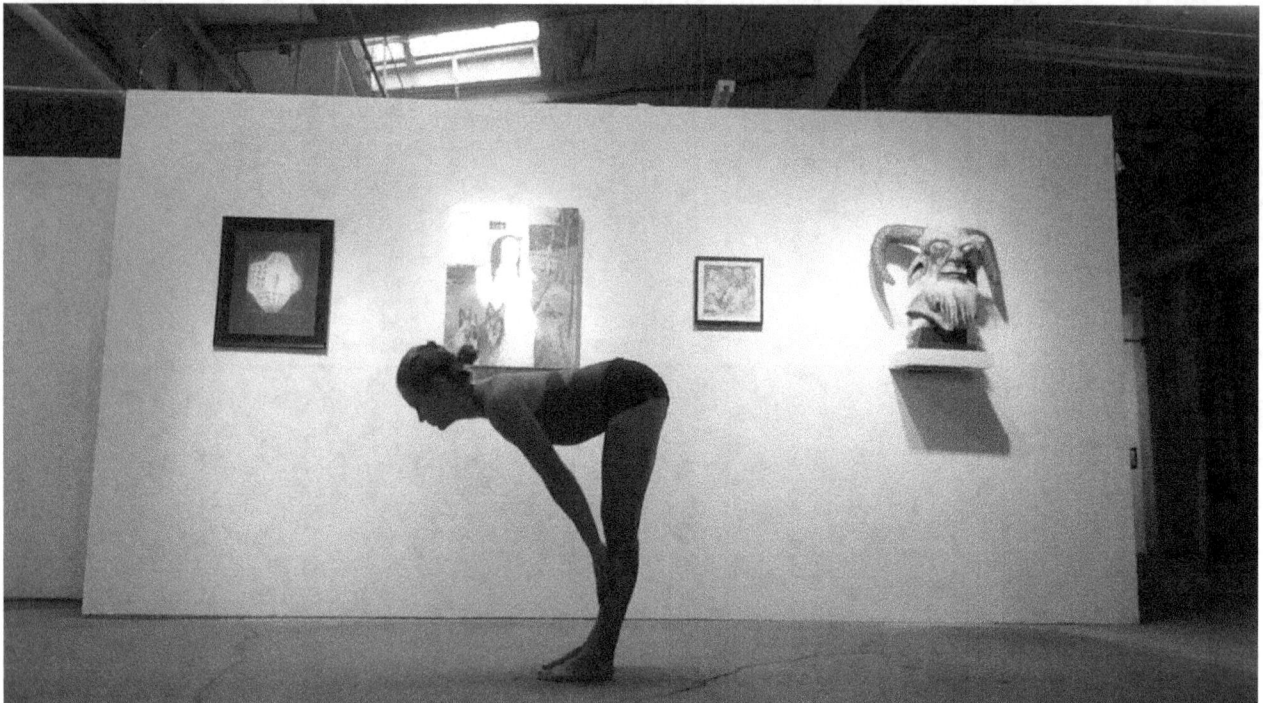

5. Exhale and step back to a high plank or straight into Four Limbed Staff Pose / Half Push-Up (*Chaturanga*). Plant the hands under the shoulders, gaze forward to keep the head from dropping, and keep your elbows tucked into your ribs to work the triceps! Make sure the body is in a straight line. Modify by dropping the knees (but not the hips) while your press down.

6. Inhale into Upward Facing Dog (*Urdhva Mukha Svanasana*), a great stretch for the back muscles and shoulder girdle. To challenge your strength, try to hover from the previous posture into this one without letting any part of your body touch the floor. Keep the shoulders and arms strong, the chest broad, the abdominals zipped in, and the legs engaged. Modify by dropping the hips and taking a cobra pose instead.

7. Exhale into Downward Facing Dog (*Adho Mukha Svanasana*). Hold for 3-5 breaths.

8. Bend your legs and look forward as you exhale.

9. Step forward to your half lift position as you inhale.

10. Exhale and fold deeper into your body.

11. Inhale as you reach your arms up to come to standing

12. Exhale as the arms come down by your sides or to your heart in prayer position.

13. Repeat 3-5 times

Sun Salutation B (Surya Namaskar B)

Sun Salute B is a continuation of Sun Salute A adding Chair Pose and Warrior 1.

It will continue to warm up the body, including the legs and the hips. Here is how you can add in the additional poses:

1. Stand in Mountain Pose
2. As you inhale, bend the legs and lift the arms into Chair Pose
3. Exhale and fold forward
4. Inhale to your half lift position
5. Exhale to step back into high plank and lower into the half push up
6. Inhale to lift up into cobra or upward facing dog
7. Exhale and press into downward dog
8. As you inhale, step your right foot forward into Warrior 1. Traditionally, you will immediately take the next exhale down into a vinyasa; however, when you are first learning, feel free to take a few breaths here to connect to the posture.
9. On your next exhale, move through Chaturanga and continue into cobra or Up dog as you inhale. Finish in downward dog.
10. Inhale and repeat the Warrior 1 on the left side. Finish the vinyasa in downward dog.
11. Take 3-5 breaths in downward dog
12. Exhale to bend the legs and look forward
13. As you inhale, step your feet to your hands and lengthen the spine.
14. Exhale to fold deeper.
15. On your next inhale, sink the hips and reach the arms up again into Chair Pose.
16. Exhale to finish with the arms by the sides or in prayer at the heart.

Suggested Sequence

1. Start seated and connect to your breath. Take as much time you need here.
2. Fold forward from seated
3. Roll up and twist to the right
4. Change the cross of your legs and repeat on the other side
5. Swing the legs around and come into Child's Pose for 5 breaths
6. Move forward into Sphinx Pose for 3-5 breaths
7. Child's Pose- 3 breaths
8. Cat/Cow- 6 rounds
9. Downward Dog- 5 breaths
10. Ragdoll Forward Fold
11. Mountain Pose- 3 breaths
12. Side Crescent Pose- 5 breaths each side
13. Sun Salutation A x 3
14. Chair Pose- 5 breaths
15. Warrior 1- 5 breaths each side
16. High Lunge for 5 breaths followed by Revolved High Lunge for 5 breaths. Repeat other side.
17. Warrior 2 for 5 breaths followed by Extended Side Angle for 5 breaths. Repeat other side.
18. Triangle Pose- 5 breaths on each side
19. Standing Leg Extension- 3 breaths to the front and side. Repeat other side.
20. Wide Legged Standing Forward Fold- 5 breaths
21. Tree Pose- 5 breaths each side
22. Staff Pose- 5 breaths
23. Seated Forward Fold- 5 breaths
24. Head to Knee Pose with the left leg extended first for 5 breaths. Then, pick up the right knee and cross into Seated Twist into the right side for 5 breaths. Repeat on the other side.

25. Boat Pose x 2- 5 breaths each
26. Bridge Pose- 5 breaths
27. Reclined Twist- 10 breaths each side
28. Savasana- 5 minutes

How to Meditate

Meditation is a great way to end a yoga practice. Practicing meditation after Savasana is a very effective method. A simple meditation you can follow utilizes your breath. Read on to learn a basic meditation.

1. Find a quiet spot and sit comfortably
2. Begin just as you would when centering to begin a practice
3. Notice the state of your mind and the state of your breath. If your mind is full of thoughts or racing at all, you breath may be shallow or disconnected. If you mind is more clear, your breath may be more deep and full.
4. Take 10 deep breaths to clear your mind. Count each inhalation and exhalation as 1. Use your mind to count, hearing it internally. This will help to focus your mind if you have an excess of thoughts.
5. After 10, breaths notice the state of your mind again. If it is more clear, continue your meditation for as long as you like. If it is still cluttered, repeat the 10 breaths until you feel more relaxed.

Start slowly with your meditation. You can begin with 5 minutes and work your way up to an hour. Be patient with yourself and allow for progress to occur slowly over time.

Tips for Practicing Yoga

1. Do not push past your edge. Take it slowly so that you do not injure yourself. Ease into the postures and use your breath to find the depth of your stretch instead of forcing anything.

2. Keep a loving attitude toward yourself as you practice. Accept your strengths and weakness with grace.

3. If anything hurts, come out of it immediately. Try to modify with props if you have not already to see it will help correct any issues in the body.

4. Do not judge yourself as good or bad- keep an open mind about where you are and how you progress in your practice. Every day is different from the previous or next. Do not hold attachments to where you are in your practice.

5. Do not eat for 1-2 hours before practicing yoga. This way you are not digesting food while you are practicing and have any unpleasant reactions.

6. Create an intention for your practice. It can be as simple as merely accomplishing a few Sun Salutations, adding one pose on to your practice a day, or finding happiness in a posture. This allows us to incorporate meaningfulness in our actions both on and off the mat.

7. Find yoga DVDs, books, or online courses that may supplement your home practice

8. Try to practice 3-5 times a week to receive the most benefit

9. Never skip Savasana. Corpse Pose is important because it allows for relaxation in the body and mind to occur after the practice. It is in this place that true union may be experienced without effort. Even if you are in a hurry, give yourself time for a short Savasana.

10. Take time to reflect after your practice. It may be as simple as a meditation or even journaling about your experience. Know that your practice is limitless and does not stop when you step off the mat. Bring it into your life!

Finding a Yoga Class

Once you feel ready to attend a yoga class, there are many options you can choose to find one. Many yoga studios today offer beginning yoga sessions in 4-8 week increments. To find a yoga studio near you, search online by typing in your location. If you choose not to sign up for an incremental session, you can also check the studio's schedule for a class such as "Yoga Basics" or something similar of that nature that you can drop in to. This may be beneficial in the beginning to find a teacher that you enjoy and resonate with.

It is important when researching yoga studios to look through the studios history and the teachers' biographies. You want to look for teachers who are at least 200 hour certified through Yoga Alliance or have done extensive study in a lineage of teachers. It is also recommended to find a teacher with experience, although you will find many new teachers as the popularity of yoga rises in the West.

If you have been practicing a beginner yoga sequence on your own for quite awhile, you may find or feel that you are ready for the next step. In this case, you have several options. Some studios may offer workshops or transitional classes to help you prepare to advance your practice. Otherwise, it is recommended to look into how a particular studio may categorize the levels of their classes. Some studios may be "all levels" and in this case, it is important to look at how long a class is. When you are first starting to practice, 1 hour is sufficient. However, some classes will be one and half hours long. This means that you will be covering more postures or spending more in depth time on particular ideas. If you are unsure about a particular class or level, reach out and contact the studio to make sure it will be a good fit for you.

Many studios will offer class levels 1-3, or even clearly labeled Beginner, Intermediate, and Advanced. Always read the class description when signing up for a class. Additionally, other class styles that may be good appropriate for beginners include Restorative Yoga, Slow Flow Yoga, or Yin Yoga. These are slower types of yoga that include longer holds of the postures.

The Benefits of Attending a Yoga Class

Attending a public yoga class is beneficial on many levels. First of all, you will have a teacher who is there to help and support you. Many teachers are trained in hands on adjustments. If you are misaligned or ready to move deeper into a posture, a teacher can physically adjust your body into the correct place or move you deeper than you thought possible.

Additionally, taking a yoga class will create a sense of community for you. By practicing in a space with others, you can share a common interest that connects you with other people. When you are surrounded by those who share a similar mindset with you, you can be further encouraged to continue along your path.

Tips for Taking Class

1. Always speak to the instructor if you have any injuries or limitations. This way they can offer you modifications and be sure not to adjust you physically in a way that may be harmful. If you do not want to be physically touched, let the teacher know as well.
2. Turn off your cell phone.
3. Take your shoes off outside of the studio space.
4. Do not be late. If anything arrive early- especially if it is your first class at a new studio. You will likely have to fill out some paperwork. Give yourself plenty of time to get set up. It's no fun to rush to a yoga class!
5. Grab any props that you may need.

6. Keep your practice appropriate for yourself. If your eyes wander to what someone else is doing, do not let it affect you. Do not judge them if they are modifying and do not try to imitate an advanced variation until you are ready.

7. Do not leave early. If you must, let the teacher know and be sure to take a Savasana on your own. It is distracting to the other students to leave early, so do not make it a habit.

Conclusion

The accessibility to learn and practice yoga today is changing lives worldwide. You can begin to benefit from a yoga practice today. The moment you begin to practice, a journey toward health and happiness begins. It begins with your decision to make positive choices in your life. Yoga can bring joy and abundance into your life, and teach you a way of living gratitude. Practicing yoga will also help you live in harmony with your community, yourself, and the planet we all live on.

When you begin to practice yoga, you will feel the way it improves not only your flexibility and strength, but also your overall health. Yoga is truly a science aimed at healing, improving, and connecting our internal bodies with our external. This connection allows you to live a resilient, and active life. There is nothing stopping you from creating the life you deserve through yoga. Start today and enjoy its benefits for life.

I Need Your Help!

Please take a minute out of your busy schedule to leave a review.

Your review will let readers know what to expect and what you liked about this book. I am looking forward to reading your review.

Thank you so much for your feedback!

How to Submit a Review

To submit a review:

1. Make sure you are signed in.
2. Hover over **Your Account** in the upper right hand corner.
3. Click on **Your Orders**.
4. Click on **Digital Orders**.
5. Click **Write a customer review** in the Customer Reviews section.
6. Rate the item and write your review.
7. Click **Submit**.

How to submit a review from your Kindle device

Please follow the link below for instructions.

http://www.dummies.com/how-to/content/posting-an-amazon-book-review-from-your-kindle.html